The Metabolic Typing ® Diet Cookbook
for 2-O, Fast Oxidation

by Nancy Dale, C.N.

Metabolic Type® and Metabolic Typing® are Registered
Trademarks of Healthexcell

Credits

contents

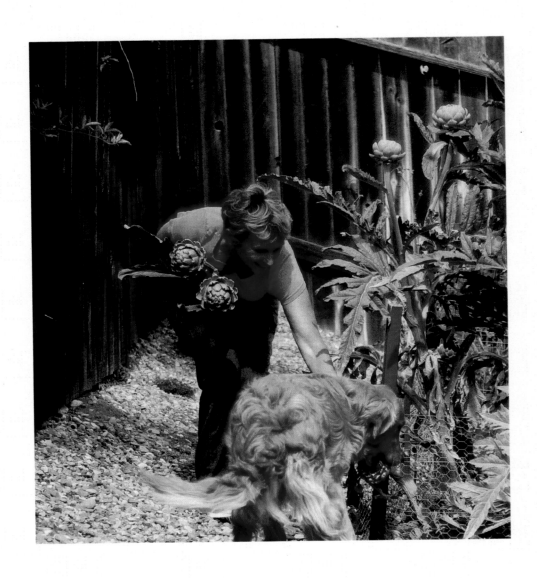

Eating to live, not living to eat.

Preface

This book took over fifteen years to create and I believe it is still a work in progress. I began cooking when I was a small girl. When I became a certified nutritionist I decided to delve into cooking from a health standpoint. Just as I completed my chef certificate in 1994 my mother was diagnosed with liver cancer. I quickly moved in with her and began cooking as a means to bring her back to health. She was given just weeks to live. I lived with her for 5 ½ years cooking all the while.

At that same time I started my clinical nutrition practice. I could only work part time while attending to my mother. I started cooking for my clients to show them what healthy meals taste like and before long I had developed a business of creating healthy meals, delivered to my clients. I lived in the Southern California area and began working with the movie industry. I was hired to work with the stars when their role required them to lose weight or to get healthier. Most of the meals in this book were created at that time.

Since moving to the Santa Barbara area I no longer cook and deliver my food. I now teach cooking classes in my home twice a year and operate two nutrition offices.

I became a Certified Metabolic Typing ® Advisor five years ago and began creating menus based on that same principle.

All of the recipes in the book have been created with your health in mind. We can not expect restaurants or prepared foods to give us health. It is my hope that you begin to love cooking as much as I do.

Bon appétit!

Nancy Dale, C.N.

Foreword

Over 30 years ago, my sojourn with Metabolic Typing® first began. From the very first encounter, I knew in my heart, in my whole being, that I had been blessed with the good fortune to have found something very special. So intriguing, so rewarding has that three decades long journey been, that nothing has been able to entice my one-pointed attention away from my quest to uncover the wondrous and amazing secrets of health possible through Metabolic Typing®.

As might be imagined, a lot can happen over three decades – or over half a lifetime in my case. And so it has. Just like the accidental discovery of a piece of a broken pot can lead to an anthropological dig that unearths an entire ancient city, what began as a one dimensional concept to determine individual dietary requirements has evolved, one discovery at a time, into an 11 dimensional model for the science of optimal health known as Metabolic Typing®.

The complexity, depth and breadth of this scientific discipline is staggering, when understood in its entirety. And yet, the day-to-day application of the truths revealed through Metabolic Typing® is utterly simple, once you know exactly what to do and how to do it.

Through the Metabolic Typing® Cookbooks, Nancy Dale has provided what may indeed be *the* most important tool for successfully living the "metabolic typing lifestyle." Nancy's hard won and heartfelt contribution to all of us in the form of the Metabolic Typing® Cookbooks is a natural expression of that rare, priceless combination of time, talent and experience, combined with a giving nature and a loving heart.

The world is rife with so-called experts. These days, anyone can write a book, self-publish it on the internet and with a little marketing savvy, appear authoritative. But the truth is that which lasts longest. And it is as true today as it has been since time immemorial, that expertise is possible only from the knowledge and understanding born from experience. Nancy Dale has an abundance of both.

Nancy has been one of the most active Certified Metabolic Typing® Advisors in the world over the last 5 years and her thriving, extremely successful practice with hundreds of enthusiastic, happy clients is testament to her expertise. Nancy's background as a successful, professional chef, combined with her extensive clinical experience with Metabolic Typing® makes her uniquely qualified to author these cookbooks. We are all fortunate to have them, myself included!

Read them. Use them. And enjoy the energy, well-being and good health that surely will ensue!

William L. Wolcott
Author, The Metabolic Typing® Diet (Doubleday, 2000)
Winthrop, Washington, December, 2009

Acknowledgement

This has been the most rewarding project I have ever worked on. This book along with the other five metabolic typing ® cookbooks has been a labor of love.

The bulk of the recipes were created from teaching my cooking classes throughout the years. It was not until 2009 that I actually fine-tuned the recipes to have only the ingredients for each particular type for each recipe-not an easy task when you consider each recipe must be created using only those ingredients.

A special thanks to Meg Fish for her amazing photography and her special artistic touch seen throughout the books; neither one of us had ever edited or created a book before so it was a pleasure to have someone so full of energy and enthusiasm to work with.

I would also like to acknowledge Bill Wolcott for his wonderful support and encouragement. Without him we would not have this incredible metabolic typing ® approach to health.

To all my students and clients who have tasted my recipes and to all of you who are about to try them; I hope you like them as much as I do.

Eating to live, not living to eat.

Nancy Dale

Introduction

These recipes are meant to be a starting point; adding more or less of any of the proteins, fats and carbohydrates until you feel satisfied. Experiment; this is how I created these recipes with the intent of customizing to fit your needs.

Most of the recipes are for multiple meals. I actually cook on Sunday for all week. I choose what recipes I am going to make and create a shopping list of ingredients a day or two prior to cooking. I involve everyone in the fun of choosing what they would like to eat. On the week-end I reserve a couple of hours to cook all of the meals for the upcoming week.

When the food has cooled, I divide each portion so that each person has the right amount to begin with.

It is a complete delight for me to walk into my kitchen at the end of a long day and open my refrigerator to any number of meals I have made that can be easily re-heated in the oven or on the stove top. In minutes we are sitting down to a great home cooked meal. This can also be very important if you have multiple Metabolic Types® in one family.

I generally steam different vegetables that can be eaten by all as well. When I am making poultry I try to have dark meat as well as breast meat.

Having multiple meals at your finger tips will help to keep everyone eating the right foods for their Metabolic Type ®.

- If you have food sensitivities omit the offending food that you have reactions to or substitute with another food from the same macronutrient group. Example: Instead of asparagus use cauliflower. Instead of salmon use halibut.

- If you have weight issues try to eat less at each meal by a mouthful or two. Wait twenty minutes and see if you are comfortable. This is what I call **"mindfully under eating"**.

- Eat sitting down at a table without distractions from the TV or computer. Never eat standing up or in your car.

- Do not eat if you are really stressed. Instead have a glass of water relax for a few minutes and wait until you have calmed down.

- Sweeteners such as stevia can be exchanged for xylitol, maple syrup, organic pure cane sugar or fruit juice, but use less of them and taste for sweetness, (less is better). You may substitute honey only in the dishes that do not require cooking, such as the yogurt or protein smoothies.

- Remember after each meal or snack you should feel satisfied, have great energy, have a sense of feeling renewed and restored. You should not have food cravings or a desire for more food. If you have any bad reactions such as feeling full, but still hungry or hyper, jittery you need to make sure you ate the right amount of protein, fats and carbohydrates for your type. An example of this might be at breakfast eating eggs makes you sluggish. Try having a protein smoothie and see if that makes you feel more energized. **This is what this whole process is about.** Learning exactly what fuel works in each body at each meal. For additional help please contact your Metabolic Typing ® advisor to help you fine-tune this process.

Glycemic Index

Corn bread	110
Instant rice	91
Corn chips	72
Millet	71
Corn tortilla	70
Corn meal	68
Rye crackers	68
Taco shell	68
Couscous	65

French baguette	95
Pretzels	81
Kaiser roll	73
Bagel	72
White bread	70
Melba toast	70
Whole wheat	69
Rye	65
Croissant	67

Linguine	55
Cheese Tortellini	50
Macaroni	45
Spaghetti	44
" " whole wheat	37

Gatorade	78
Cranberry juice	68
Coca cola	63
Orange juice	55

Yogurt with fruit	36
Milk (fat free)	32
Cottage cheese	24

Watermelon	72
Pineapple	66
Cantaloupe	65
Raisins	64
Apricot	31

Grains

Stoned wheat thins	67
Quick Oats	65
Basmati white rice	58
Whole wheat pita	57
White rice	56
Corn	55
Oatmeal, old fashioned	48
Bulgur	48
Barley	25

Bread

Hamburger bun	61
Cheese pizza	60
Bran muffin	60
Blueberry muffin	60
Pita	57
Sourdough	54
Oat bran	54
Banana	47
Pumpernickel	41

Pasta

Vermicelli	35
Spaghetti	35
Fettuccini	32
Spaghetti(protein enrich)	28

Beverages

Grapefruit juice	51
Pineapple juice	48
Apple juice	41
Tomato juice	38

Dairy

Yogurt	14
Whole milk	30

Fruit

Orange	43
Grapes	43
Strawberries	40
Apple	36
Pear	36

Papaya	60	**Fruits, Cont.**	
Banana	53	Peaches	28
Kiwi	52	Plum	24
Date	50	Grapefruit	25
		Cherries	22
Potato	104	**Potato**	
Red potato	93	Mashed potato	73
Instant mashed	83	Potato chips	54
French fries	76	Sweet potato	54
		Yam	51
Pea soup	66	**Legumes**	
Split pea and ham	66	Lima beans	32
Black beans	54	Chick peas	32
Butter beans	36	Navy beans	31
Black eyed peas	42	Lentils	30
Garbanzo	34	Kidneys	23
Beans (string/green)	0	Peanuts	13
Cashews	22	**Nuts**	
Almonds	0	Macadamia	0
Brazil	0	Pecans	0
Hazelnuts	0	Walnuts	0
Carrots	92	**Vegetables**	
Beets	64	Eggplant	0
Tomato	15	Snow peas	0
Mushroom	0	Artichoke	0
Broccoli	0	Peppers	0
Cauliflower	0	Asparagus	0
Cabbage	0	Zucchini	0
Celery	0	Cucumber	0
		Lettuce	0
		Meat/Protein	
Beef	0	Lamb	0
Chicken	0	Pork	0
Eggs	0	Fish	0

Try to keep most of your choices below "40".

Facts on Fiber

What does fiber do? There are two types of fiber: insoluble (the kind found in vegetables, wheat and whole grains) and soluble (the kind found in fruits, oats, barley and legumes).

Insoluble fiber seems to fight cancer by binding to or diluting cancer-causing agents in the gut and speeding them through the colon.

Soluble fiber has its own part to play in keeping the body healthy: preventing heart disease. This kind of fiber forms a gel in the intestines that traps and ushers cholesterol out of the body. Soluble fiber can help reduce insulin levels, which in turn lowers triglycerides.

High fiber diets slow down the rate of digestion, which lowers both blood sugar levels and the insulin needed to transport that blood sugar into the cells.

Foods high in soluble fiber stay in your stomach longer creating a feeling of fullness that lasts longer so you eat less. Eating a diet high in soluble fiber will allow you to lose an average of 1/2 pound per week.

Food	Fiber (grams)
wheat-bran cereal (1/2 cup)	11
oatmeal (1 cup cooked)	4
brown rice (1 cup)	3.5
barley (1/2 cup cooked)	3
whole wheat bread	2
potato (baked with skin on)	5
carrots (1/2 cup cooked)	3
Brussels sprouts (1/2 cup cooked)	2.5
black-eyed peas (1/2 cups cooked)	8
black beans (1/2 cup cooked)	7.5
kidney beans (1/2 cup cooked)	6.5
lima beans (1/2 cup cooked)	6.5
apple (with skin on)	4
pear (with skin on)	4
raisins (2/3 cup seedless)	4
raspberries (1/2 cup)	4
orange (1 medium)	3.5

Boosting your fiber intake to the recommended 25-35 grams a day is good for your health. It can cause excess gas and be tough on your stomach. Here are some tips to ease the discomfort.

Go slowly. Increase your fiber by 5 grams per week.

Think small. Eat smaller portions of problematic foods such as beans and whole grains. Eat fruit that contain insoluble fiber which are easier to digest.

Emotional Eating

You are continually nourished by the world around you. When you close yourself to that nutrition, you feel the need to provide it yourself.

That is when food becomes magnetic. You do not have the capacity to provide yourself with the nourishment that you crave, and so eating becomes endless. **It is not the calories you seek, but contact with your soul (going home) and with the universe.** That is where true satisfaction exists, and is complete, nourishing and sustains life. No amount of chocolate, chips, salsa, or macaroni and cheese can substitute for this.

You can not receive too much nourishment from the universe any more than you can breathe too much air. When you do not have enough air, you gasp. When you do not have enough nourishment for your soul you seek substitution in food. You can eat too much food.

Eating more than you need is not necessarily a sign of a chemical imbalance or eating the wrong types of food. It is a sign that you are fundamentally out of balance. Until that correction is made, compulsive hunger will continue to remind you that you have inner work to do. It is a gift; gentle reminders to pay attention to what is going on in your world and make the corrections to create a healthy body, mind and spirit.

Dieting and exercise cannot reach the root of obsessive eating. Eating the right foods in the right amounts and exercising are prerequisites for physical health. However, illnesses are symptoms of deeper dynamics that bear directly on the purpose of your life and where you are accomplishing it.

Eating is Sacred. Every time you eat or drink anything, say to yourself, "Eating is sacred. I eat this food to nourish my body."

When you emotionally eat you deprive yourself from learning about your emotions. Next time you go for the cookie when you have had a **"bad"** day consider sitting down and reflecting on the events of the day and see what you can learn from this.

What is more worthy of your attention—a gift of knowledge about yourself or a cookie?

The Protein Type Diet

Strong Appetites-You may feel the need to eat frequently, even after a meal or snack. Overeating can be a problem.

Cravings for Fatty, Salty Foods-If you begin to eat rich fatty foods with carbohydrates such as pizza with sausage, you will find yourself craving sugar; the more you eat the more you want.

Failure with Low-fat Low Calorie Diets-Losing weight by counting calories does not work for you. Eating good quality protein along with vegetables and healthy fats does work.

- **Focus on protein** and fat at every meal or snack along with vegetables or your preferred fruits (but eat those sparingly).
- **Purine-containing foods** are best for your type. These are oxidized (converting to energy) at the proper rate for your metabolism.
- **Snack as needed.** Make sure your snacks are protein and fat rich. Stay away from the carbohydrate snacks.
- **Be very cautious of grains and high starch carbohydrates.** They convert to sugar very quickly in your system leaving you wanting more.
- **Fruits do not do well in most protein types.** They should be eaten at the end of the meal and in small amounts.
- **Eat fats and oils.** These satisfy you as long as they are pure. Stay away from partially hydrogenated, margarines and trans-fats. Eat organic butter raw if possible along with cold pressed oils.
- **Avoid alcohol.** Caffeine, Sugar, Fruit juices and High Glycemic Foods.
- **Avoid foods high in gluten.** Eat Manna bread or soured sprouted breads if you must eat bread.

Food Menu's for Protein type #2-O

Breakfast

Protein smoothie with and added raw egg or
Almond Pancakes with1/4 cup fresh fruit with1/2 cup full fat yogurt and 2 T. nuts or
1-2 Eggs (poached, fried, hardboiled or scrambled), Canadian bacon with fruit, or
Sausage Mushroom Spinach Frittata with zucchini muffin, or
Salmon Omelet with cottage cheese and blueberries, or
Mini Mushroom and Sausage Quiches with Nancy's No-carb zucchini muffin

Lunch

Artichoke and Ripe Olive Tuna Salad on Avocado or
Stuffed artichoke with Crabmeat Salad, or
Chicken and Spinach Soup with Fresh Pesto, or
Split Pea and Ham Soup, or
Meatloaf with sautéed vegetables, or
Salmon Chowder with a piece of manna bread and butter

Dinner

Pork tenderloin with Green Beans with Pecan or
Chicken Enchiladas and a big green salad, or
Nancy's spiced greens with turkey sausage, or
Stacked Salmon and spinach, or
Rolled Chicken Stuffed with Vegetables and Broiled Cauliflower
Mushroom and spinach squash, or
Meatloaf and Mashed Cauliflower "Potatoes" or
Bison Steak with Prosciutto wrapped Asparagus

Snacks

2 T. hummus with celery
2 T. peanut butter or almond butter and an apple or celery
1-2 hard boiled eggs
¼ cup nuts or energy trail mix
Pear with string cheese

Shopping List for #2-O

Green = Ideal (eat these foods at every meal)
Black = For variety (but emphasize 'Ideal' foods)
Italics = Caution (eat only rarely)

Protein

Heart or Kidney
Chicken Breast
Chicken thighs and legs
Organic whole chicken
Turkey (dark)
Beef (grass fed)
Canadian bacon
Bacon
Buffalo
Rabbit
Lamb
Elk
Frozen fish
Halibut
Sea Bass
Shrimp
Crab
Mahi-mahi
Red Snapper
Salmon
Abalone
Scallops
Sardines
Tuna
Turkey sausage
Chicken sausage

Vegetables

Celery
Bok Choy
Carrots
Salad greens
Cauliflower
Kale
Spinach
Avocado
Mushrooms
Asparagus
Corn
Green Peas
Beet
Zucchini
Sweet potato
Yam
Jerusalem artichoke
Green beans
Olives
Fennel
Jicama
Kohlrabi
Radish
Eggplant
Daikon
Fresh parsley
Artichokes
Potatoes (Russet)
Split peas
Lettuce (all)

Fruits

Apples
Pears
Coconut
Bananas
Apricot
Nectarine
Kumquat
Plum
Cherries
All berries
Rhubarb
Peach

Dairy

Plain yogurt (full fat)
String cheese
Colby
Swiss (full fat)
Cheddar (full fat)
Jack (full fat)
Provolone
Gouda (full fat)
Goat feta
Proserum® Whey
Organic Chicken eggs
Organic Duck eggs
Cream
Butter
Raw butter
Parmesan
Romano
Roquefort
Swiss

Grains

Spelt
Wild Rice
Buckwheat
Oats
Amaranth
Triticale
Brown rice
Quinoa
Barley

16

Oils & Dressings

Olive oil
Sesame oil
Walnut oil
Ranch Dressing
Cilantro Dressing

Nuts & Seeds

Brazil nuts
Hazelnuts
Flax
Hickory nuts
Macadamia nuts
Peanuts
Pecans
Pumpkin seeds
Walnuts
Almonds
Pistachios
Sesame seeds
Cashews
Chestnuts
Poppy Seeds
Sunflower Seeds

Condiments, Spices

Vegetable broth
Chicken broth
Coconut milk
Almond milk
Peanut butter
Almond butter
Bread crumbs
Soy sauce
Sea salt
Pepper
Ginger
Oregano
Thyme
Basil
Coriander
Cumin
Dill
Fennel
Tarragon
Turmeric
Paprika
Cayenne
Stevia
Xylitol
Agave
Honey
Apple cider vinegar
Wasabi
Mayonnaise
Maple Syrup
Nutmeg
Saffron
Vanilla
Chocolate

Legumes

Adzuki beans
Black beans
Fava beans
Great northern beans
Lentils
Mung beans
Red beans
Tempeh
Garbanzo beans
Navy beans
Pinto beans
White beans
Black eyed peas

Nancy's No-Carb Zucchini Muffins Pg 54

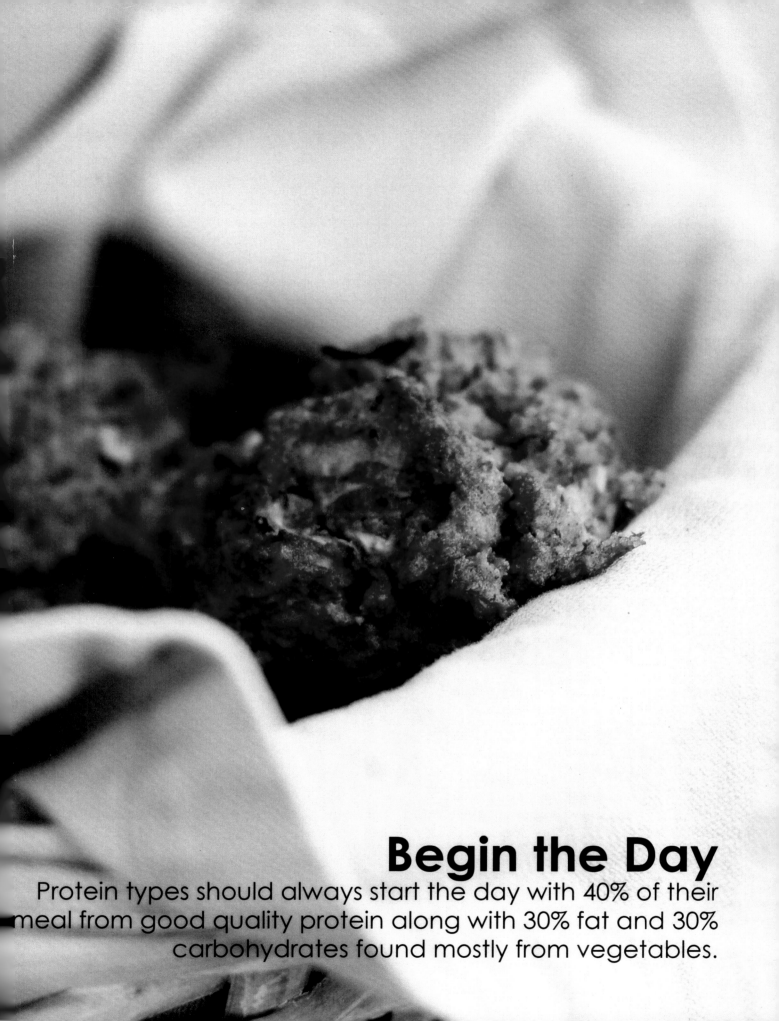

Begin the Day
Protein types should always start the day with 40% of their meal from good quality protein along with 30% fat and 30% carbohydrates found mostly from vegetables.

Protein Smoothies

Serves one each recipe (may add raw egg for more protein)

1	**Basic Berry-**Combine milk, with frozen fruit and scoop of protein powder in blender. May add ground nuts or LSA* if desired for extra fiber.	1-1 ½ C. organic milk or almond milk ½ C. frozen fruit **1 scoop Goatein, hemp or egg white protein powder 1-2 T. nuts (see below recipe for LSA)*
2	**Creamy Monkey-** Mix milk, protein powder, peanut or almond butter, frozen banana and blend.	1-1 ½ C. organic milk or almond milk **1 scoop Goatein, hemp or egg white protein powder 1 T. peanut or almond butter ½ frozen banana
3	**Reese's Pieces-** Same ingredients as creamy monkey but add organic cocoa powder.	Use 1 T. cocoa powder to above recipe for Creamy monkey.
4	**Tropical Delight-**Combine milk with coconut milk, frozen banana, pineapple with protein powder; blend until smooth. May add nuts or LSA* mix if needed for more fiber.	1 C. organic milk or almond milk ½ C. coconut milk ½ frozen banana 1/3 C. frozen pineapple **1 scoop Goatein, hemp or egg white protein powders 1-2 T. nuts (see below recipe for LSA)*
5	**Raspberry Delight-**Blend protein powder, frozen raspberries with cocoa until smooth. May add LSA* mix.	1-1 ½ C. organic milk or almond milk 1 scoop Goatein, hemp or egg white protein powder ½ C. frozen raspberries 1 T. cocoa (optional) 1-2 T. nuts (see recipe below for LSA)*
6	***LSA nut mixture** Mix and grind until fine using a coffee grinder. Can be stored in refrigerator for 3 months.	3 C. organic flaxseeds 2 C. organic raw unsalted sunflower seeds 1 C. raw unsalted organic almonds

*May use ground flax seed or flax seed oil

** Goatein, hemp or egg white are different types of protein powders. Select one that not have added sugars. Add the correct amount of scoops according to directions on container to make a smoothie with approximately 18-30 grams of protein.

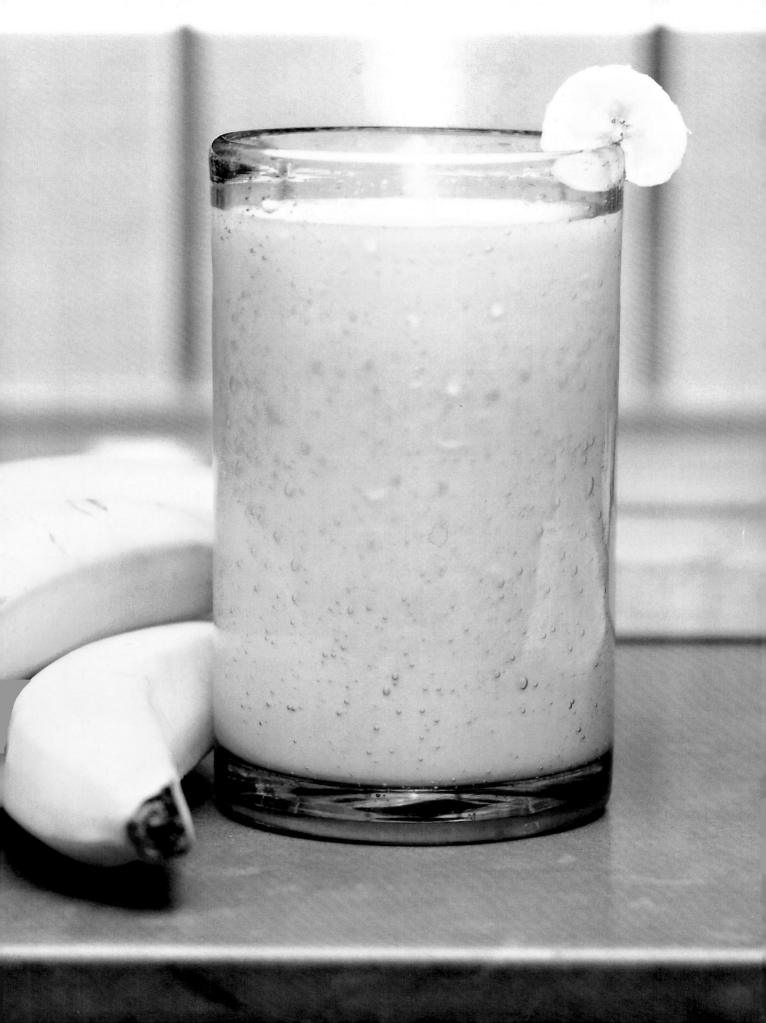

Sausage Mushroom Spinach Frittata
(Calories: 350, 35 g protein, 12 g fat 25 g carbohydrates)

Serves 6

#	Instructions	Ingredients
1	Preheat oven to 400° F	
2	Oil pie or quiche pan and sprinkle with almond meal; set aside.	1 T. olive oil ¼ C. almond meal(may substitute bread crumbs)
3	In a skillet melt butter and add mushrooms cooking 3-4 minutes on medium flame. Slice the sausages and add to mushrooms and cook 2-3 minutes. (If using pork, cook 6-8 minutes and add to mushrooms).	1-2 T. raw organic butter 4 oz. mushrooms, sliced 8-12 oz. pre-cooked turkey or chicken sausages (may use pork sausage)
4	Steam the spinach leaves 2-3 minutes and squeeze out any moisture. Add to mushroom mixture.	4-6 oz. of organic spinach leaves
5	Mix together in a bowl. Beat until well mixed.	¼ C. raw cream 10-12 organic eggs
6	Place mushroom mixture in pan and add feta cheese. Top with parmesan cheese.	4 oz. feta cheese ¼ C. parmesan
7	Pour egg mixture over all.	
8	Bake for 30 minutes.	

Mini Mushroom and Sausage Quiches
(Calories per two muffins: 225, 18 g protein, 13 g fat, 10 g)

Makes 10-12 minis

1	Preheat oven to 325° F	
2	Heat skillet over medium flame. Add sausage and cook 6-8 minutes. Drain and transfer to a bowl and let cool 5 minutes	8 oz. turkey or pork sausage, removed from casing and crumbled into small pieces
3	Add oil to the skillet and cook mushrooms stirring often until golden brown about 5-7 minutes. Transfer to the sausage bowl and let cool 5 minutes. Stir in spinach, feta and pepper.	1-2 t. olive oil 8 oz. mushrooms, sliced ½ C. spinach, cooked and drained ¼ C. goat feta cheese ½ t. black pepper
4	Whisk in a bowl the eggs and milk until frothy. Divide the egg mixture evenly among the oiled and foiled muffin cups. Place a heaping tablespoon of the sausage mixture into each cup.	8 eggs 1 C. whole raw milk foil muffin liners 1 T. olive oil
5	Bake until the tops are just beginning to brown, about 25 minutes.	
6	Individually wrap in plastic for up to 3 days or freeze up to 1 month.	

Asparagus and Mushrooms over Eggs

(Calories: 200, 8 g protein, 12 g fat, 10 g carbohydrates)

Serves 2-3

1	Slice asparagus into ½ inch pieces and heat in oil adding mushrooms sautéing until tender crisp about 8 minutes; set aside	1 lb. asparagus, trimmed 1 T. olive oil ½ lb. mushrooms, trimmed
2	Add more oil and sauté celery for 4-6 minutes or until soft. Add to asparagus.	2 T. olive oil 1 celery stalk, chopped fine
3	Scramble or poach eggs and place one or two on each plate. Place mixture over eggs and sprinkle with cheese. Serve immediately.	4-6 eggs ¼ C. Swiss, grated ¼ t. sea salt ¼ t. pepper

Tip: You will need some extra protein like a slice of ham or a buffalo burger to make this a complete meal.

24

Almond Pancakes

(Calories per pancake: 125, 6 g protein, 8 g fat, 6 g carbohydrates)

Serves 2

1	Mix ingredients together and cook as you would other pancakes. They will not bubble, so turn when side becomes light brown.	1 C. almond meal 2 free-range eggs ¼ C. water ¼ C. chopped apples 2 T. coconut oil 1 T. stevia, may use ¼ t. maple syrup ½ t. cinnamon ¼ t. salt
2	Serve with pat of butter and chopped walnuts and sliced bananas	butter walnuts banana

Tip: These pancakes should be served with eggs or another protein to be balanced.

Banana Coconut Flour Nut Muffins
(Calories: 184, 12 g protein, 8 g fat, 16 g carbohydrates)

Makes 12 muffins

1	Preheat oven to 350° F	
2	Mix coconut flour and baking powder in a separate bowl; set aside.	1 C. coconut flour* 1 t. baking powder
3	In a mixing bowl, beat eggs gradually…. Add milk, stevia, coconut oil, butter, vanilla and salt.	6 organic free range eggs 2 T. organic milk 1 T. stevia (substitute ¼ C. maple syrup) 2 T. coconut oil* (warmed to liquid) 2 T. organic butter ½ t. vanilla 1/8 t. sea salt
4	Mash the bananas and add to the egg mixture. Continue mixing and slowly add the flour mixture and walnuts and mix until blended.	2 green tipped bananas ½ C. walnut pieces
5	Oil and fill muffin cups with batter.	
6	Bake for 20 minutes.	

*Purchase at www.tropicaltraditions.com

Salmon Omelet
(Calories: 250, 24 g protein, 13 g fat, 8 g carbohydrates)

Serves 2

1	Preheat oven to 350° F	
2	Separate egg yolks and lightly beat, set side. Combine the 4 egg whites in a small mixing bowl and beat until light and fluffy; add egg yolks and salt and pepper to taste.	2 large eggs and 2 egg whites ¼ t. sea salt ¼ t. pepper
3	Lightly oil an oven proof skillet and place over medium heat. Spread the egg mixture in the pan and cook for 3-5 minutes until the bottom is light brown.	1 T. coconut oil or butter
4	Place the skillet in the hot oven on the middle rack and bake 3 minutes. Dot with goat cheese, salmon and parsley and bake 1 more minute.	3 oz. goat cheese 3 oz. smoked salmon (or left over salmon)
5	To serve fold the omelet in half.	

Nancy's No-Carb Zucchini Muffins
(Calories: 170, 7 g protein, 14 g fat, 2 g carbohydrates)

Makes 18 small muffins

1	Preheat oven to 350° F	
2	Grate. Set aside.	3 C. zucchini
3	Chop. Set aside.	1 C. walnuts
4	Sift into a bowl… … and then add the grated zucchini and chopped walnuts	2 C. almond meal ½ C. egg white protein powder 1 t. baking soda 2 t. cinnamon 1 t. ground ginger 1 t. ground nutmeg ¼ t. ground cloves ¼ t. salt
5	Mix together in another bowl.	3 eggs, slightly whipped ¼ C. maple syrup 1 t. vanilla 1/3 C. coconut oil ¼ C. apple juice
6	Pour wet mixture into dry mixture and mix well (You may need a little extra apple juice to make a soft batter).	
7	Spoon into a small muffin tin.	Bake for 20-25 minutes.

28

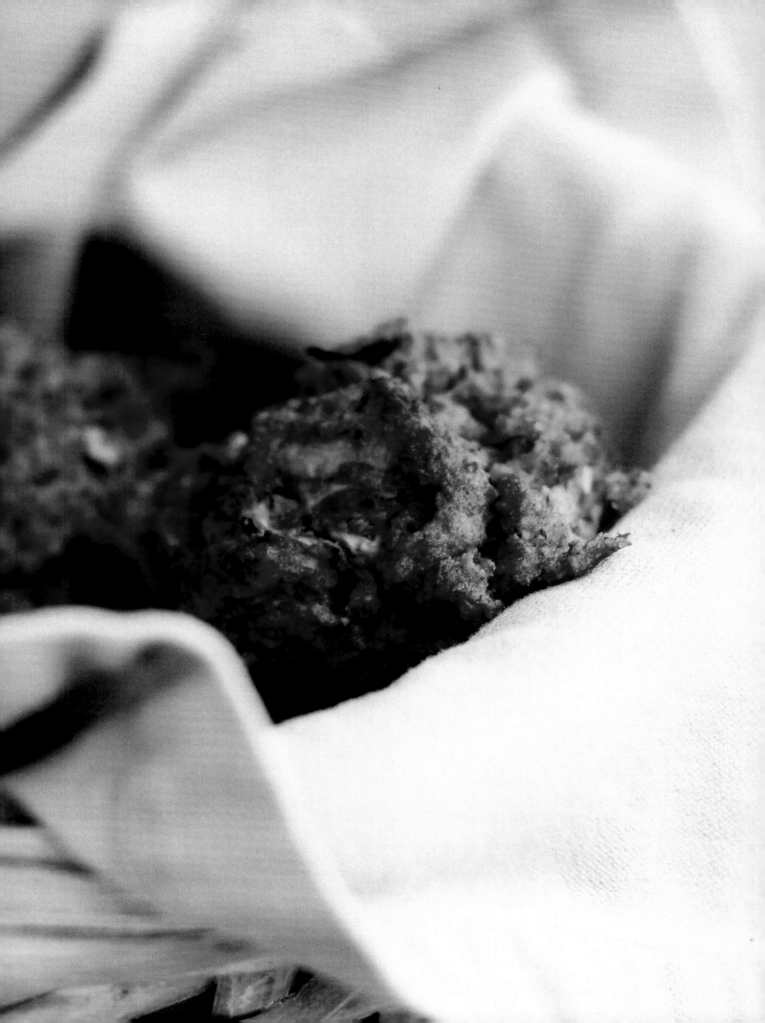

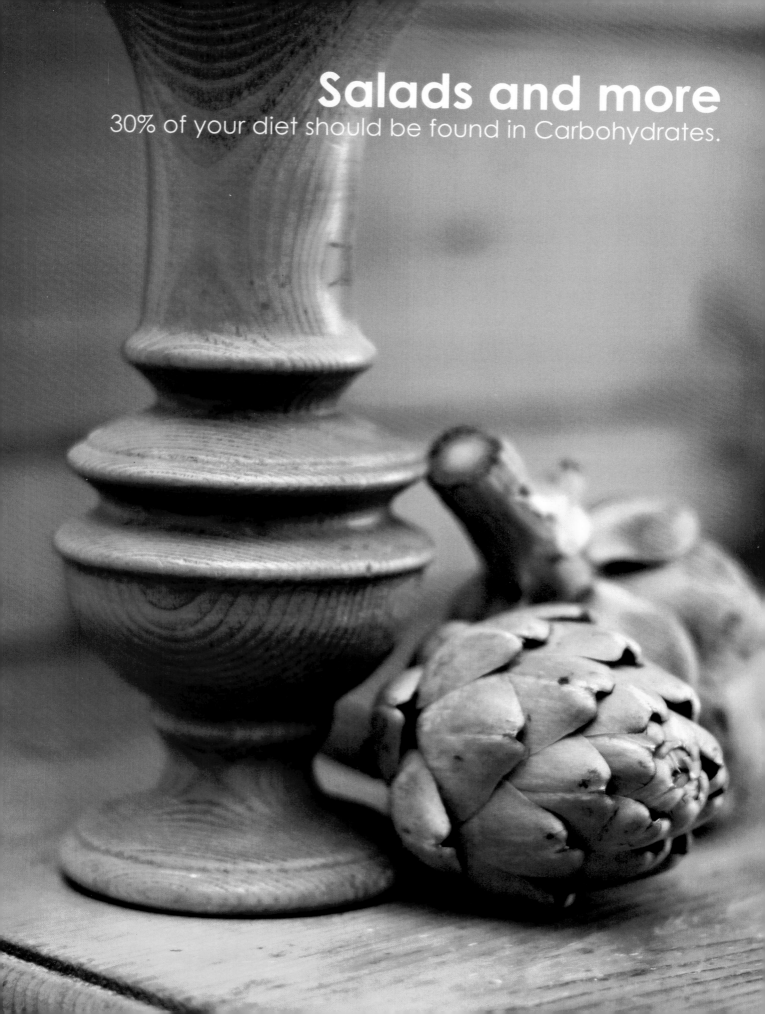

Salads and more

30% of your diet should be found in Carbohydrates.

Cold Asparagus with Sesame-ginger Vinaigrette
(Calories: 150, 2 g protein, 11 g fat, 10 g carbohydrates)

Serves 4

1	Mix dressing together and chill.	2 T. apple juice 2 T. olive oil 1 t. grated fresh ginger 2 t. tamari wheat free soy sauce 1/8 t. stevia (may use ½ t. maple syrup) ¼ t. toasted sesame oil
2	On a bed of spinach leaves place chilled cooked asparagus and pour dressing on top.	1 lb. asparagus, trimmed, steamed and chilled 1 bunch of fresh cleaned spinach leaves

Tip: This makes a great appetizer. Be sure and add protein with this like Chicken Crusted in Almond or the Grass-Fed Beef recipes if using as a side dish.

Artichoke and Ripe Olive Tuna Salad On Avocado
(Calories: 270, 20 g protein, 24 g fat, 12 g carbohydrates)

Serves 5

1	Combine ingredients in a bowl.	1-12 oz. can or 2-6 oz. cans tuna in olive oil 1 C. chopped artichoke hearts ½ C. chopped olives ¼ C. mayonnaise 1 ½ t. chopped fresh oregano or ½ t. dried ¼ t. sea salt ¼ t. pepper
2	Place Boston lettuce on salad plate with ¼ avocado. Place 1/5 of the tuna salad (¾ cup) on each avocado. Serve immediately.	5 Boston lettuce leaves 2-3 avocados, peeled and quartered

Tip: This makes a great lunch as is.

Stuffed Artichoke with Hot Crabmeat Salad
(Calories: 290, 32 g protein, 10 g fat, 20 g carbohydrates)

Serves 4

1	Trim the artichokes and steam for 30 minutes.	4 artichokes
2	While the artichokes are steaming heat the oil and butter in a large skillet and sauté celery and carrots for 2 minutes and then add the mushrooms; cook 5 minutes.	1 T. olive oil 1 T. butter 1-2 stalks celery, finely chopped 1 large carrot, finely chopped ½ lb. mushrooms
3	Add the cooked rice, shellfish and water chestnuts, cooking until heated through about 5 minutes.	1½ C. brown rice, cooked 1 lb. crab meat, cooked 1 lb. small shrimp, frozen precooked ½ C. water chestnuts
4	Toss in almonds.	¼ C. almonds, sliced
5	Remove the center section of each artichoke and stuff each with the rice mixture. Serve hot or cold.	

Spinach Salad
(Calories: 380, 30 g protein, 18 g fat, 26 g carbohydrates)

Serves 2 large or 4 small

1	Place eggs in saucepan and add enough water to cover them. Bring to low boil and then reduce heat to medium low for 10 minutes. Pour off the hot water and run under cold water to cool them. Once cooled peel the eggs and chop them.	8 free-range eggs 1 qt. water
2	Mix ingredients together. ...set aside Cook the bacon and crumble; set aside	3 T. walnut oil (may use olive oil) 1 T. blue cheese, crumbled ¼ t. sea salt ¼ t. pepper 4 slices pork bacon
3	Toss the spinach with ½ the dressing and place on the salad plates. Top with chopped eggs, bacon, carrots and pecans. Drizzle with the remaining 2 tablespoons dressing.	6 C. baby spinach, cleaned and dried 1 C. carrots, shredded 2 T. pecans, toasted and chopped

Tip: To toast nuts or seeds: Cook in a small dry skillet over medium–low heat, stirring constantly, until fragrant and lightly browned about 2-4 minutes.

Chicken and Spinach Soup with Fresh Pesto Pg

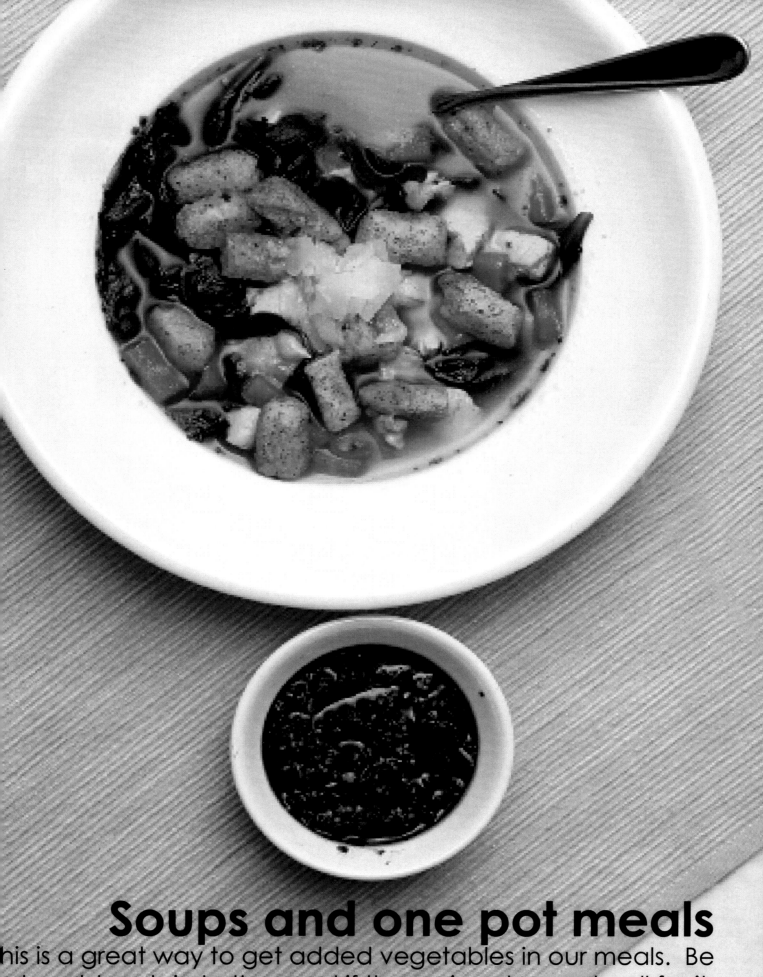

Soups and one pot meals

his is a great way to get added vegetables in our meals. Be
e to add protein to the meal if the recipe does not call for it.

Cleansing Broth
(Calories per cup 70, 2 g protein, 3 g fat, 9 g carbohydrates)

Makes 1 ½ quart

1	Steam or boil the sweet potato for 10 minutes.	1 medium sweet potato, peeled and quartered
2	In a 4 quart pan add water, squash, cabbage, spinach and celery and cook for 8 minutes.	1 qt. filtered water 1-2 yellow squash 3-4 oz. cabbage, chopped 4 oz. spinach leaves 3-4 stalks celery, chopped
3	Add sweet potatoes to the pan.	
4	Puree in blender adding the olive oil, tamari and milk.	1-2 T. olive oil 1-2 T. tamari wheat free soy sauce 1 C. whole organic raw milk
5	Serve immediately. May be refrigerated and reheated or enjoyed at room temperature or chilled.	
6	Last in refrigerator 2-3 days.	

Tip: This is a great way to get some extra vegetables in. Make sure you eat protein along with it.

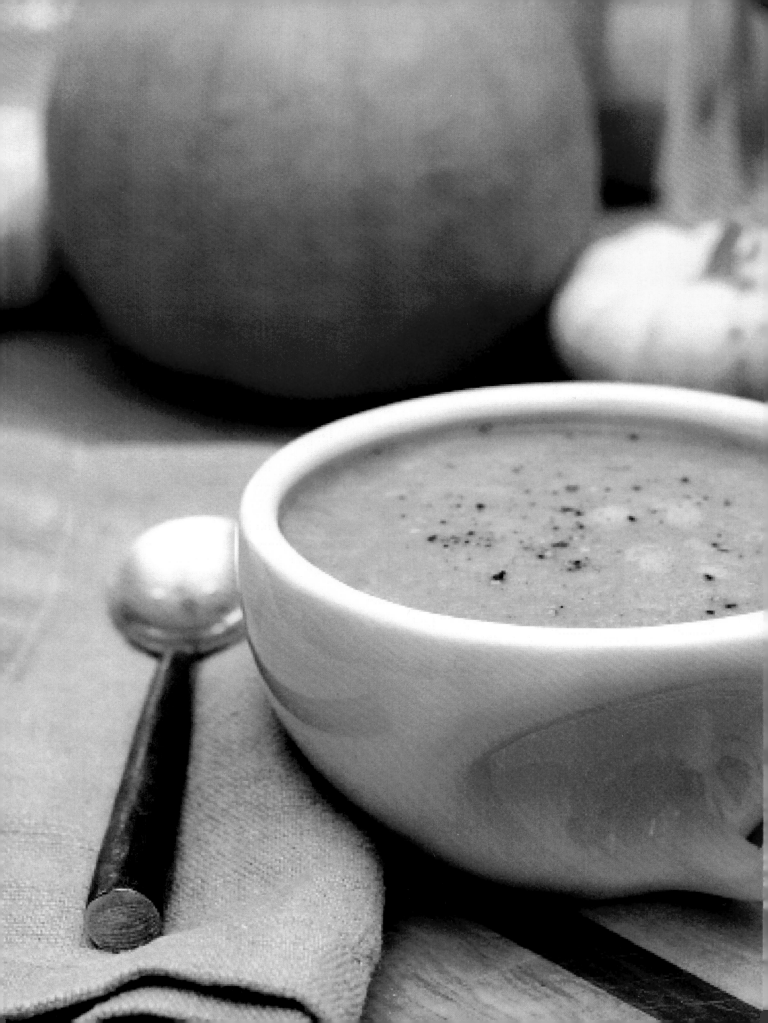

Vegetable Broth #2

Makes 1 ½ quarts

1	In a soup pan place cut up vegetables in 1 quart of filtered water and bring to a boil. Reduce and simmer about 6-8 minutes.	1 qt. filtered water 8 oz. green beans 2-4 stalks celery ½ bunch spinach leaves 4 oz. kale
2	Puree in blender adding olive oil or butter, tamari, salt and pepper and cream.	1-2 T. olive oil or raw butter 1 T. organic tamari, wheat free soy sauce ¼ C. raw organic cream or milk ¼ t. sea salt ¼ t. pepper
3	Place in air tight container; may be stored in refrigerator for 2-3 days.	

Tip: Having this on hand can help you get your vegetables in while eating your protein. Example: For breakfast try a cup of this broth with two eggs fried in butter and a couple slices of bacon.

Tip: I have heated this up on the stove and added an egg or two stirring it while it heats. Taste great and gives you good energy while not feeling full.

Chicken Bone Broth

Makes one pint

1	Place bones in a large pot and cover with water and add the vinegar. Let stand for one hour.	1 pastured organic chicken, bones only 2 qts. filtered water 2 T. apple cider vinegar
2	Bring the pot to a simmering low boil and remove any foam scum that appears on the top of the water. Continue simmering on low boil for 24 hours.	
3	Remove bones and place in a container. Use or freeze for later use.	

Salmon Chowder

(1 ½ cup serving: 115, 30 g protein, 5 g fat, 14 g carbohydrates)

Serves 4-6

1	Heat oil in a large saucepan over medium heat. Add carrots and celery and cook 3-4 minutes until vegetables are just brown.	1 T. olive oil 1/3 C. carrots, chopped 1/3 C. celery, chopped
2	Add broth, water, salmon, cauliflower and chives and bring to a simmer. Cover and cook until the salmon is done about 8 minutes.	4 C. chicken broth 1½ C. water 2 12-oz. skinned salmon fillet (wild caught) 3 C. cauliflower florets, chopped 3 T. fresh chives chopped or 1 ½ T. dried chives
3	Remove the salmon to a clean cutting board and flake into bite size pieces. Add potatoes, dill or tarragon and mustard into the soup and blend.	1½ C. leftover potato, cubed ¼ C. fresh dill, chopped or 2 t. dried tarragon 1 T. Dijon mustard
4	Return soup to a simmer. Add the salmon. Season with salt and pepper.	¼ t. sea salt ¼ t. pepper

Tip: If you are using potatoes that are not cooked, cube them and add them to the broth and water and cook 20 minutes before adding the salmon in step 2.

Chicken and Spinach Soup with Fresh Pesto
(1 ½ cup serving: 284, 28 g protein, 8 g fat, 16 g carbohydrates)

Serves 6

1	Heat the oil in a large Dutch oven over medium heat. Add the carrots and the chicken; cook turning the chicken and stirring frequently about 3-4 minutes.	2 t. olive oil ½ carrot, chopped 6-8 chicken thighs, boned and skinned
2	Add broth and marjoram bring to a boil and then reduce to a simmer for 5 minutes.	5 C. chicken broth 1 ½ t. marjoram, dried
3	With a slotted spoon take the chicken out and cut into bite size pieces.	
4	Add spinach and beans to the soup and bring to a low boil for 5 minutes.	6 oz. baby spinach leaves 1 15-oz. can great northern beans, rinsed
5	In a food processor combine oil, parmesan cheese, and basil. Process until course paste forms adding water if necessary.	1 T. olive oil ¼ C. parmesan cheese, grated 1/3 C. basil leaves, fresh
6	Stir chicken into soup along with the pesto made from the food processor.	
7	Season with pepper. Heat until hot.	¼ t. pepper

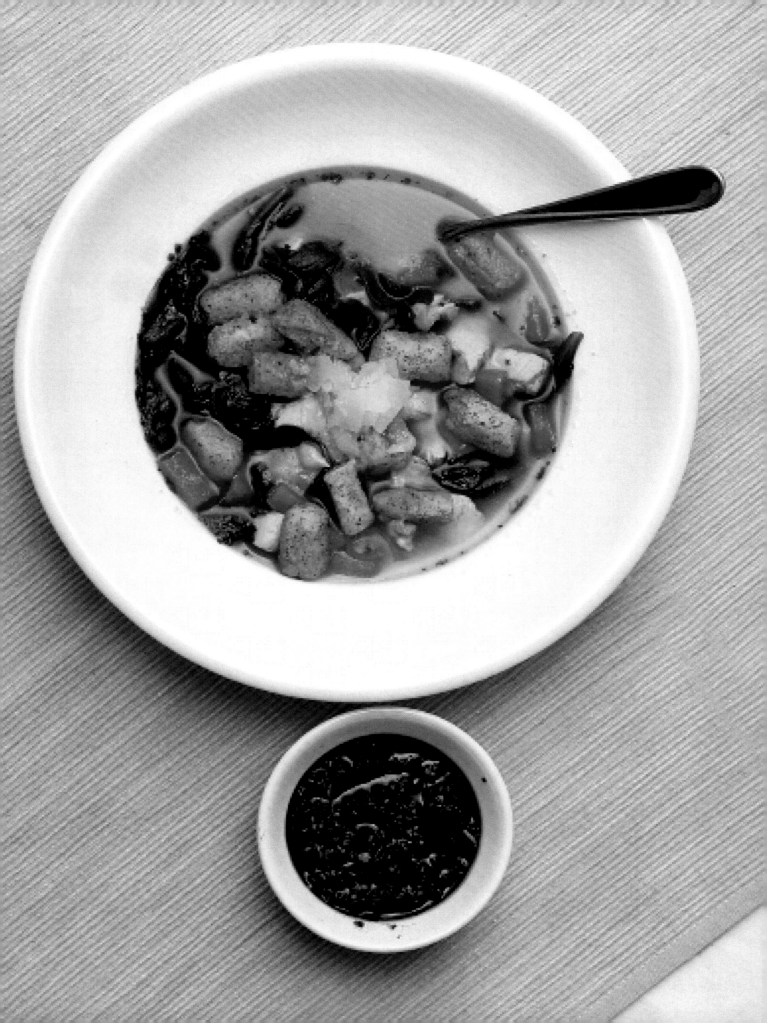

Mushroom Barley Soup (with beef)
(Calories: 200, 9 g protein, 10 g fat, 20 g carbohydrates)

Serves 6-8

#	Instructions	Ingredients
1	In a 5-6 quart Pot add oil and butter; sauté celery and mushrooms for 5 minutes; Add tamari sauce and basil and cook 1 minute.	1 T. olive oil 2 T. raw butter 2 C. celery, diced 1 lb. mushrooms, sliced ¼ C. tamari wheat free soy sauce 1 t. basil, dried
2	In another sauté pan add oil and cook beef until done. Add to the pot with the water and barley cover and simmer 30 minutes, stirring occasionally.	1 T. olive oil 1 lb. beef (ground or tenderloin) shredded 8 C. filtered water ¾ C. barley
3	Dice the cauliflower into bite size pieces and add to soup and cook another 15 minutes.	1 small cauliflower, diced
4	Reduce heat and add peas and simmer until just hot.	10 oz. frozen peas
5	Adjust seasonings to taste and serve.	¼ t. sea salt ¼ t. pepper

Tip: This soup should be served along with more protein like a pot roast or roasted chicken.

Split Pea with Ham Soup
(Calories: 328, 38 g protein, 4 g fat, 35 g carbohydrates)

Serves 6-8

#	Instructions	Ingredients
1	In a large soup pot heat oil and add carrot, celery, apple and cilantro. Reduce heat and add spices sautéing and stirring often until vegetables are done about 10 minutes.	1-2 T. olive oil 1 large carrot, chopped 2 stalks celery, trimmed and chopped 1 green apple, chopped ¼ C. cilantro leaves, chopped 1 T. curry powder 2 t. ground cumin 2 t. whole mustard seeds 1 t. coriander 1 t. ground turmeric
2	Stir in split peas and water to cover them by two inches. Bring to a boil and then reduce heat and cover; simmer one hour or whenever the peas are soft and ready to puree.	1½ C. split peas 1½ qt. filtered water
3	Puree with an immersion blender or in a food processor. Return to pot.	
4	On low heat stir in ham. Season with salt and pepper.	16 oz. ham, cooked, diced ¼ t. sea salt ¼ t. pepper
5	Serve hot. May be refrigerated 2-3 days.	

Green Beans with Pecans Pg 49

Vegetables and more
30% of your diet should come from these.

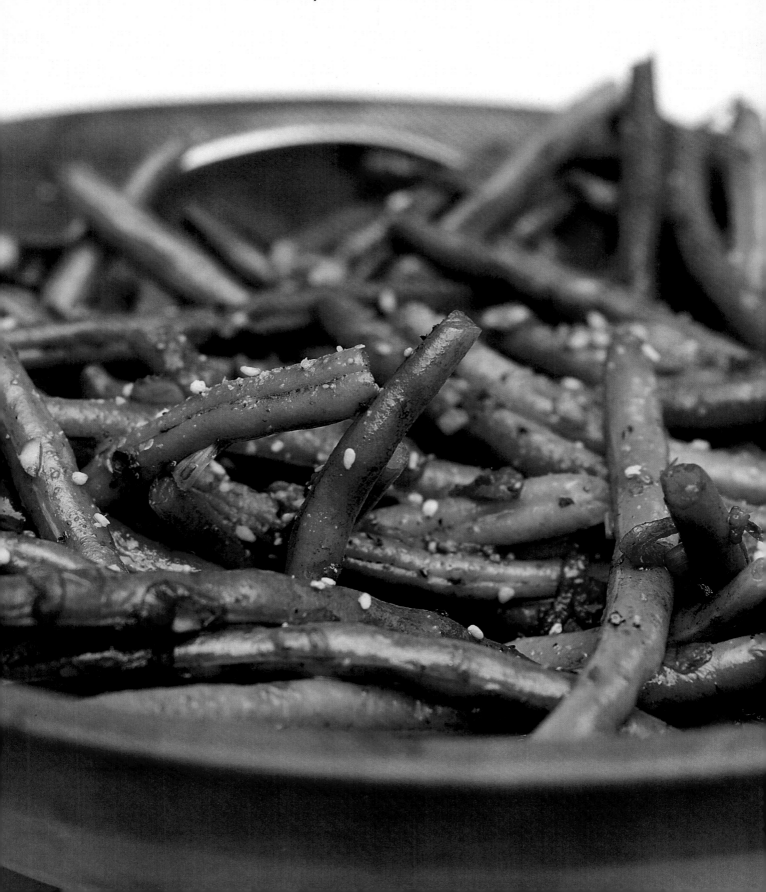

Prosciutto wrapped Asparagus
(Calories: 39, 3 g protein, 15 g fat, 3 g carbohydrates)

Serves 4

1	Preheat grill to medium.	
2	Toss asparagus with oil, salt and pepper in a medium bowl.	16 spears of asparagus cleaned and trimmed 1 T. olive oil or walnut oil ¼ t. sea salt ¼ t. pepper
3	Wrap 1 length of prosciutto around the middle of 4 asparagus spears.	2 very thin slices prosciutto cut in half lengthwise
4	Grill the asparagus in bundles turning once or twice until done about 10 minutes. Serve immediately.	

Tip: This makes great appetizers.

1. Restaurant Green Beans
2. Green Beans with Pecans
3. Green Bean Pate with Basil

1	In a large pot of water add salt. (The salt sets the color and you rinse it off with cold water). Bring salted water to a rolling boil, put in green beans and cook 6-8 minutes. Rinse and drain on paper towel. Use in salads or add butter and serve.	1 lb. fresh green beans cleaned and trimmed. 1 qt. water 1 T. sea salt
2	Cook beans until tender about 6 minutes. Meanwhile, heat oil and butter in a pan and sauté celery until softened. Stir in savory. Add the beans and pecans, season with salt and pepper and serve.	1½ lb. green beans cleaned and trimmed 2 T. organic butter 1 T. olive oil ¼ C. fresh celery, chopped ½ t. savory, dried 1 C. pecans ¼ t. sea salt ¼ t. pepper
3	Steam the beans about 6 minutes. Using a food processor, process the beans, eggs, pine nuts, basil and vinegar until roughly pureed. Remove from bowl and mix in just enough mayonnaise to hold mixture together. Stir in salt and pepper to taste. Chill.	½ lb. fresh green beans, cleaned and trimmed 1 T. olive oil 3 hard boiled eggs ½ C. pine nuts 1 t. vinegar (apple cider) 3 T. fresh basil, chopped 1-2 T. mayonnaise ¼ t. sea salt ¼ t. pepper

49

Tip: These are side dishes to be used with main course of protein.

Green Beans with Mushrooms

(Calories: 120, 2 g protein, 10 g fat, 6 g carbohydrates)

Serves 4

1	Brown the mushrooms in the butter; about 4 minutes.	2 T. raw butter ¾ lb. mushrooms, sliced
2	Clean and blanche the green beans in salted water for 30 seconds. Drain.	1 lb. green beans cut into 2 inch lengths
3	Add the chicken broth to the mushrooms and onions and bring to a boil. Add paprika, dill and salt and pepper to taste. Boil for 5 minutes.	1 C. chicken broth ¼ t. paprika ¼ t. dill, dried ¼ t. sea salt ¼ t. pepper
4	Add the green beans and sour cream. Simmer on low for 8-10 minutes and serve.	½ C. sour cream

Tip: Side dish to be served with a nice grass fed steak or piece of wild caught fish and a green salad.

Blue Cheese-Walnut Green Beans
(Calories: 163, 6 g protein, 12 g fat, 10g carbohydrates)

Serves 4

1	Clean, trim and cut diagonally into 1 inch pieces. Steam for 6-8 minutes. Transfer to a bowl and add olive oil, salt and pepper and toss.	1 lb. green beans 1 T. olive oil ¼ t. sea salt ¼ t. fresh ground pepper
2	Toast the walnuts until light brown but not burnt about 2 minutes.	1/3 C. walnuts, chopped
3	Toss the green beans with blue cheese and sprinkle each serving with the walnuts.	1/3 C. blue cheese, crumbled (may use gorgonzola)

Tip: This should be paired with a protein dish such as the Grass-Fed Beef recipes and perhaps a small spinach salad.

Broiled Cauliflower
(Calories: 148, 7 g protein, 8 g fat, 12 g carbohydrates)

Serves 4

1	Preheat broiler to 425° F	
2	Break a head of cauliflower into florets and steam for 6 minutes.	1 large head of cauliflower
3	Arrange the florets on a broiler pan and brush with melted butter and sprinkle with parmesan cheese and dust with paprika.	2 T. melted raw butter 1-2 T. parmesan cheese paprika
4	Broil until cheese melts and begins to turn brown. Serve immediately.	

Tip: This is an easy vegetable dish to be served with one of the protein dishes.

Cheesy Cauliflower Bake

(Calories: 75, 3 g protein, 4 g fat, 10 g carbohydrates)

Serves 4

1	Preheat oven to 350° F	
2	Steam cauliflower until tender about 8 minutes. Drain and mash using a potato masher or food processor.	1 large cauliflower, cut into florets
3	Add butter, cream, cheese and salt and pepper to taste.	2 T. butter 2 T. cream 2 T. parmesan cheese ¼ t. sea salt ¼ t. pepper
4	Place in a buttered casserole dish and sprinkle with sesame seeds and parmesan.	1 T. Gamasio (sesame seeds) 2 T. parmesan cheese
5	Bake the oven for 10-15 minutes. Serve immediately.	

Tip: Kids love this dish as it reminds them of "mac and cheese". Make sure there is protein like Rolled Chicken Stuffed with Vegetables or Chicken Crusted in Almonds.

Mashed Cauliflower "Potatoes"

(Calories: 90, 4 g protein, 7 g fat, 2 g carbohydrates)

Serves 4-6

#		
1	Steam the cauliflower until soft 6-8 minutes.	4 C. cauliflower florets
2	Puree in a food processor or mash them like you would potatoes.	
3	Add butter and cream. Season with salt and pepper. Serve immediately.	2 T. butter ¼ C. half and half or raw cream ¼ t. sea salt ¼ t. pepper

Tip: These can replace mashed potatoes easily. With a Glycemic Index of "0" compared with mashed potatoes at "73", it makes a great choice.

Cheese and Spinach Stuffed Portobello
(Calories: 201, 14 g protein, 10 g fat, 13 g carbohydrates)

Serves 4

1	Preheat oven to 450° F	
2	Coat a rimmed baking sheet with oil and place the mushrooms gill side up, sprinkled with salt and pepper. Roast for 20-25 minutes.	4 large Portobello mushrooms ¼ t. sea salt 1/8 t. black pepper
3	Mash ricotta, spinach, parmesan, olives, Italian seasoning and black pepper in a medium bowl.	1 C. ricotta cheese 1 C. fresh spinach leaves finely chopped ¼ C. parmesan cheese 2 T. Kalamata olives, finely chopped ½ t. Italian seasoning ¼ t. black pepper
4	Warm the marinara sauce on the stove until hot.	¼ C. prepared *marinara sauce
5	When mushrooms are tender, carefully pour out any liquid accumulated in the caps. Return to baking sheet gill side up. Spread ½ tablespoon of marinara sauce over each cap; mound a generous 1/3 cup ricotta filling into each of the caps and sprinkle with the cheese.	1/2 C. parmesan cheese
6	Bake until hot, about 10 minutes. Serve with the remaining marinara sauce.	

Tip: *A small amount of marinara sauce may be used although it is not one of your recommended foods. It is allowed in very small amounts to season this dish.

Enchilladas Pg 60

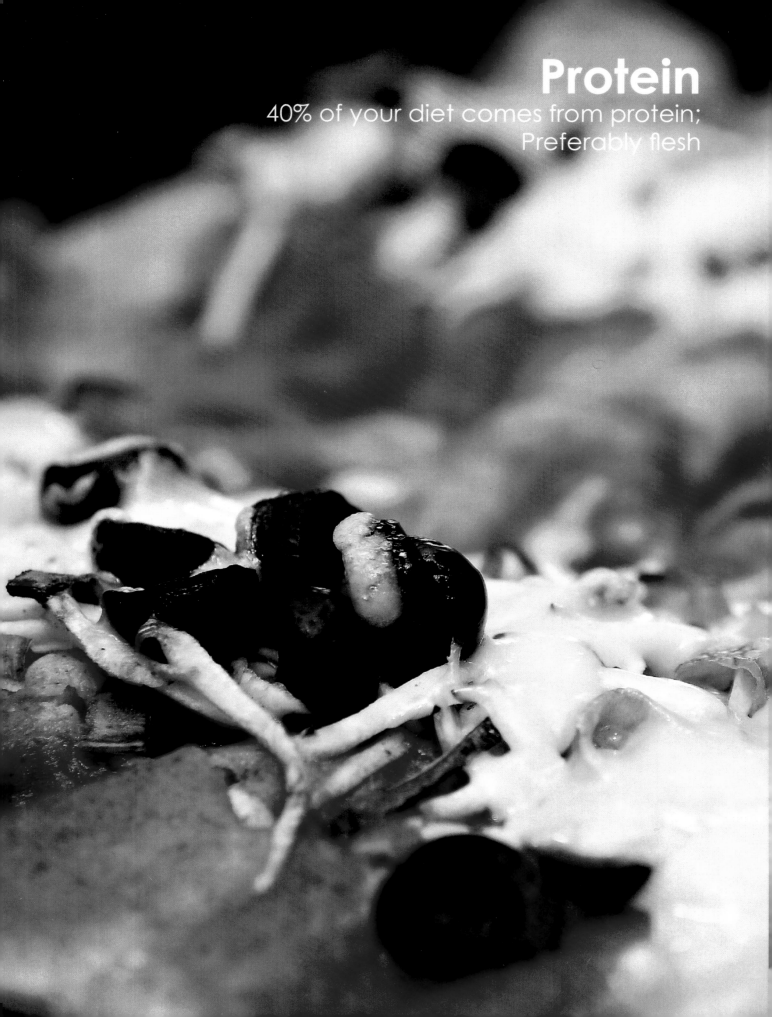

Protein
40% of your diet comes from protein;
Preferably flesh

Rolled Chicken Stuffed Vegetables
(Calories: 250, 24 g protein, 10 g fat, 16 g carbohydrates)

Serves 4

#		
1	In a small sauté pan place balsamic vinegar on medium heat and heat until liquid is reduce by ½ making a reduction; set aside.	½ C. balsamic vinegar (optional)
2	Pound the chicken between two sheets of plastic until ¼ inch thick.	4 boneless, skinless breast or thighs
3	Steam the spinach and drain all water off and pat dry.	8 oz. of spinach
4	Add water to egg and beat until frothy and place in a pie tin. In another pie tin place almond meal, salt and pepper.	1 egg ¼ C. water ½ C. almond meal ¼ t. sea salt ¼ t. pepper
5	Place ¼ of the spinach on each chicken piece along with feta cheese and roll up and secure with pick.	4 oz. goat feta cheese
6	Dip rolled chicken into egg mixture and then into almond meal. Sauté in oil for 10-15 minutes until light brown and done. Serve with balsamic reduction.	

Salmon Cakes
(Calories: 150, 17 g protein, 7 g fat, 8 g carbohydrates)

Serves 4

1	Preheat oven to 400° F	
2	In a food processor process ingredients until minced fine.	½ C. celery ½ C. bread crumbs ½ C. almond meal ¼ C. cilantro 1 egg 1 T. Tabasco sauce ¼ t. sea salt and ¼ t. pepper
3	Combine the salmon with the mixture and form into patties on waxed paper and chill for 30 minutes.	1 lb. cooked salmon, diced
4	Heat oil in skillet over medium heat. Cook the patties about 2-3 minutes per side. Transfer to oven and cook through about 4 minutes. Serve immediately.	1-2 T. olive oil or coconut oil

Tip: This can be served over a bed of lettuce for a complete light meal. Instead of citrus which is not allowed with this type add a tablespoon of apple cider vinegar, sea salt and pepper to sour cream for a dressing.

Enchiladas

(Calories: 350, 24 g protein, 10 g fat, 30 g carbohydrates)

Serves 6-8

1	Preheat oven to 375° F	
2	Sauté chicken about 5 minutes each side; shred. If using beef, brown well until done about 10 minutes; set aside	8-10 chicken thighs, skinless, boneless or 1 pound ground beef
3	Grate zucchini and set aside.	2-4 zucchini
4	Grate the cheeses; set aside.	4 oz. cheddar cheese 4 oz. jack cheese
5	Place enchilada sauce in a pan and warm.	1 large can *Enchilada sauce (Rosarita or similar)
6	Heat tortillas on the stove until warm.	12-18 corn tortillas
7	Dip the tortilla into the sauce and place in a large baking pan. Add thighs or meat, zucchini mixture and cheese in the center and roll up. Continue until all are filled.	
8	Pour remaining sauce over rolled enchiladas and sprinkle with olives and any remaining cheese. Bake for 15-20 minutes. May be frozen.	1 small can sliced organic black olives

Tip: Enchilada sauce is not on your plan but a small amount may be tolerated.

Chicken with Capers
(Calories: 160, 27 g protein, 5 g fat, 12 g carbohydrates)

Serves 4

1	Sprinkle salt and pepper over chicken.	4 chicken breast or thighs, boneless, skinless ¼ t. sea salt ¼ t. pepper
2	Heat oil in skillet over medium heat. Add chicken and sauté 6 minutes each side or until done. Remove and set aside keeping warm.	1 T. olive oil or coconut oil
3	To skillet add broth, salt and pepper and capers. Stir scraping skillet to loosen brown bits. Cook liquid until reduced to ¼ cup (about 2 minutes).	½ C. chicken broth 3 T. capers, rinsed ¼ t. sea salt ¼ t. pepper
4	Spoon over the chicken and serve.	

Tip: This goes great with a cup of Split Peas soup or Blue Cheese and Walnut Green Beans.

Chicken Crusted in Almonds
(Calories: 220, 33 g protein, 10 g fat, 2 g carbohydrates)

Serves 6-8

1	Cut chicken in half and place between two sheets of plastic and pound until ¼ inch thick or twice the original size.	6-8 boneless, skinless chicken breasts or thighs
2	Mix together the almond meal, salt and pepper and place in a pie tin.	½ C. almond meal ¼ t. sea salt ¼ t. pepper
3	In another pie tin crack an egg and whip with a small amount of water until frothy.	1 egg 1/8 C. water
4	Heat oil in a large skillet over medium flame and place the chicken dredged in egg and then almond mixture into it. Sauté each side 2-4 minutes until light brown. Serve immediately. Extras can be refrigerated for 2-3 days.	2 T. olive oil or coconut oil

Tip: This goes great with Sautéed Vegetables. Be sure to make extra for your salad the next day.

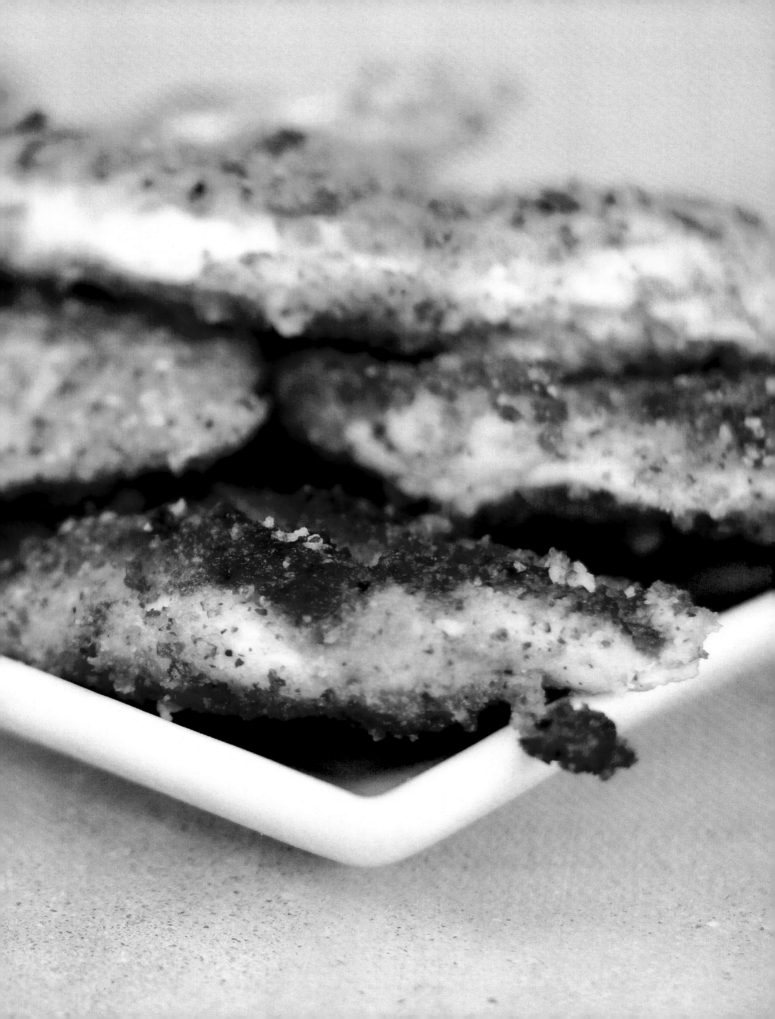

Stacked Salmon and Spinach
(Calories: 310, 24 g protein, 20 g fat, 10 g carbohydrates)

Serves 4

1	Preheat broiler to 475° F	
2	Clean, cut and steam cauliflower for 8 minutes. Puree in food processor adding butter and half and half until smooth. Season with salt and pepper. Keep warm.	4 C. cauliflower 2 T. butter 2 T. half and half (may use milk) ¼ t. sea salt ¼ t. pepper
3	Place fish on broiler pan and broil each side 4 minutes.	4 four oz. salmon fillets
4	Steam spinach leaves for 4 minutes; drain.	1 lb. spinach leaves
5	On a dinner plate place ¼ of the cauliflower in center of plate. Layer with fish and spinach and drizzle with balsamic vinegar reduction. Serve.	¼ C. balsamic vinegar reduction*

Tip: *To make balsamic vinegar reduction place ½ C. balsamic vinegar in a saucepan and with medium heat reduce liquid by ½.

Bacon-Wrapped Pork Tenderloin Filets
(Calories: 280, 22 g protein, 20 g fat, 5g carbohydrates)

Serves 6-8

1	Prepare pork: Trim off silver skin and fat and cut into 2" thick filets. Prepare the grill on medium high.	2 pork tenderloins (1 ½ lb. each)
2	To make the Chimichurri sauce; mince in food processor until smooth the first four ingredients and then add the oil, vinegar and water. Divide sauce in half to be served with meal.	2 C. cilantro leaves ½ t. pepper ½ t. red pepper flakes ½ C. olive oil ¼ C apple cider vinegar 2 T. water
3	Wrap bacon strips around each filet overlapping the ends and skewer each filet. Brush with Chimichurri sauce.	12 strips bacon, thin
4	Grill each side turning every 4 minutes basting with sauce each turn. Grill until internal temperature reaches 145° F, about 15 minutes. Serve with extra sauce.	

Tip: Served with Sautéed Vegetables or Cold Asparagus with Sesame-ginger Vinaigrette makes this a complete meal.

Bison Cooking Tips
(Per/100g raw, trimmed: 22 g protein, 2 g fat)

Use lower temperatures for cooking as Bison is extra lean.

1	**Steaks** Grill or BBQ 6 inches from heat source on medium high. Cook 4-6 minutes per side. Meat thermometer should read between 135° for rare to 145° F for medium rare.	¾ to 1 inch thick *Steaks
2	**Roasts** In oven use uncovered pan with rack. Season as desired. Cook at 275° (135°-145°F meat thermometer). Preheat BBQ and turn off one side. Place roast on side that is turned off. Cook to rare 135° F or medium rare 145° F.	Rib, Loin or Tenderloin
3	**Pot Roast and Braising** Use pan with cover to create moist heat to cook. Brown in small amounts of oil. Simmer on top of stove until done. Fork should go into meat easily.	2-3 pound *Sirloin Tip, *Inside Round, Shoulder Brisket, Ribs 1-3 T. olive oil *marinate prior to cooking 8-24 hours

Tip: *Marinade: 1½ C. olive oil, ½ C. tarragon vinegar, ½ C. water, ¼ t. oregano, dried, ¼ t. basil, dried, ¼ t. sea salt, ¼ t. pepper. Combine and pour over meat and refrigerate. This marinade works great on beef as well.

Greek Bison Burgers with Yogurt Sauce
(Calories per burger 352, 35 g protein, 12 g fat, 30 g carbohydrates)
Without bun calories 252, 35 g protein, 12 g fat, 5 g carbohydrates)

Makes 4 patties   *Preheat grill to medium high*

1	**Burgers** Place bison, spinach, feta and spices in a large bowl and gently combine without over mixing. Form into patties. Oil the grill rack to make sure they do not stick to grill. Grill on medium 5-6 minutes each side or until meat thermometer reads 135°F-145°F).	1 lb. bison ½ C. cooked spinach, squeezed and dried ½ C. feta cheese (sheep or goat) 2 t. dill, fresh, chopped 1 t. oregano, fresh, chopped 1 t. cumin ¾ t. sea salt ½ t. pepper
2	**Yogurt Sauce** Combine yogurt and spices in a small bowl. Season with salt and pepper.	¾ C. plain Greek style yogurt 1 t. apple cider vinegar 1 t. dill, fresh, chopped 1 t. mint, fresh, chopped ¼ t. sea salt ¼ t. black pepper
3	Assemble the burgers on either rolls or large Boston lettuce topped with yogurt sauce slices of cucumber.	4 Boston lettuce leaves or 4 hamburger buns 16 thin slices English cucumber

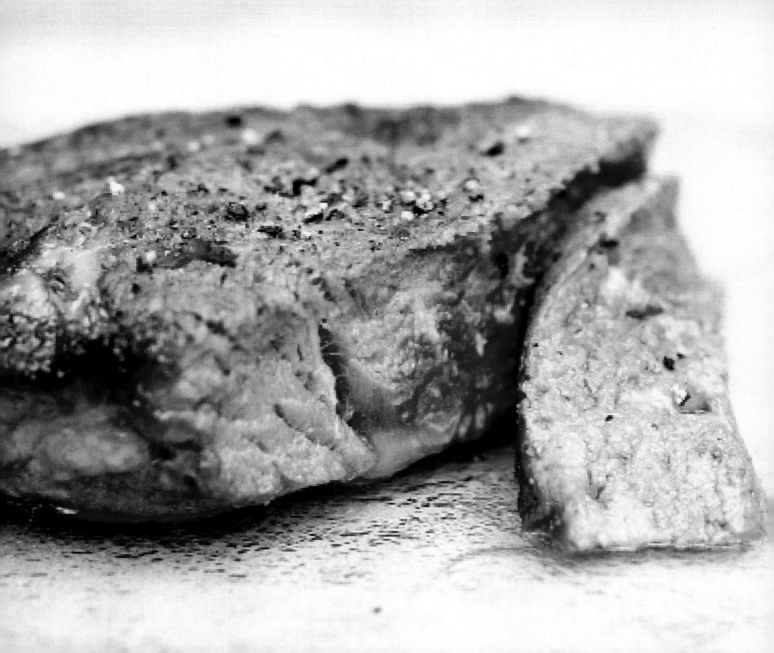

Nancy's Grass-Fed Beef Recipes

1 Baked Round Steak

Spread butter on Steak, sprinkle mushrooms over steak and salt and pepper. Wrap in 2 thicknesses of foil; place in covered roaster with rack. Bake in 325° oven for 2 hours.

Serves 6-8

¼ lb. raw butter
2 lb. round steak
4 oz. mushrooms, sliced
Sea Salt and pepper

2 Beef and Bacon Rollups

Combine all ingredients except the bacon. Make into 8 patties and surround each patty with a slice of bacon fastened with a toothpick. Broil or grill each side about 7 minutes. Serve on a Boston lettuce or a bun.

Serves 8

10 slices thin beef or pork bacon
1 free-range egg, beaten
3 T. Worcestershire sauce
2 lb. ground beef
1 C. raw cheddar cheese, shredded
1 t. sea salt
½ t. pepper

3 Beef Kabobs

In a large bowl, whisk together oil and seasonings; add beef, and vegetables, tossing. Alternately thread beef with vegetables on 12 inch metal skewers. Broil or grill about 12-15 minutes turning often.

Serves 6-8

1 pound Grass-fed Beef stew meat, cubed
1 medium zucchini, chopped in rounds
12 large mushrooms
1 T. olive oil
1 t. honey
½ t. oregano, dried
¼ t. pepper

4 Chopped Steaks in Mushroom Sauce

Combine ground beef and salt in large bowl and shape into four ½ inch patties. Heat oil in skillet and brown patties 10-12 minutes turning once. Remove from skillet; keep warm. Add mushrooms and ¼ cup of beer to skillet; cook over medium heat 5 minutes, stirring occasionally. Combine gravy mix with remaining beer in a small bowl; mix until smooth and stir into mushrooms along with the thyme. Simmer until heated through and pour over patties.

Serves 6-8

1 ¼ pound ground beef patties
¾ t. sea salt
¼ t. pepper
1 T. olive oil
8 ounces sliced mixed fresh wild mushrooms(oyster, cremini, shitake)
1 ½ C. beer (12 ounces)
1 package (.87-.88 ounce)brown gravy mix
½ t. thyme, dried or 2 t. fresh chopped thyme

5 Pot Roast with Baby Vegetables

Sprinkle roast with salt and pepper. Place carrot in the bottom of a 5-6 quart Crock Pot. Lay meat on top of the whole vegetables. Pour in the broth and Worcestershire sauce and whole herb; cover and cook on low for 5-6 hours. Remove the cover and add baby vegetables and salt and pepper cover and cook for an additional 1-1 ½ hours.

Serves 6-8

3-5 pound top beef chuck roast, trimmed of excess fat
¼ t. sea salt
¼ t. pepper
1 carrot, whole
1 C. beef broth
2 T. Worcestershire sauce
2 garlic cloves, whole(optional)
1 rosemary sprig or 1 t. dried
2 thyme sprigs or 1 t. dried
1 pound new red potatoes
1 C. baby carrots
1 C. baby squash
1 C. button mushroom, stems removed

6 Liver and Apples

Sprinkle liver with salt and pepper. Melt butter in skillet. Cook liver about 3 minutes each side. Remove and keep warm. Add apple to skillet; cook until onions are light brown. Serve over liver.

Serves 6-8

1 pound sliced beef liver
½ t. salt
1/8 t. black pepper
¼ C. raw butter
2 apples, cored , peeled and sliced

Slow/Low Heat Cooking Techniques

1	Preheat oven to 225° F	Bake 5 minutes per oz. of food
2	Using a glass roasting dish with lid, place chicken skin side up on the bottom. Place lid on securely; Bake for 1 hour and 20 minutes.	1 lb. chicken thighs, breasts or legs
3	Combine ingredients and make into four patties; place in a glass dish and put lid on; bake 1 hour and 20 minutes.	1 lb. of ground beef, turkey or bison ¼- ½ t. herbs (your choice) ¼ t. sea salt ¼ t. pepper
4	Place in a glass dish, drizzle with butter or olive oil, salt and pepper and bake covered for 1 hour and 20 minutes.	1 lb. of any firm fish (salmon, halibut, cod bass) 1 T. olive oil or butter ¼ t. sea salt ¼ t. pepper

Tip: Use this technique for vegetables as well. Place squash (whole) pierce the skin and bake 5 minutes per ounce in a glass dish with lid on.

Raspberry-Rhubarb Pie Pg 76

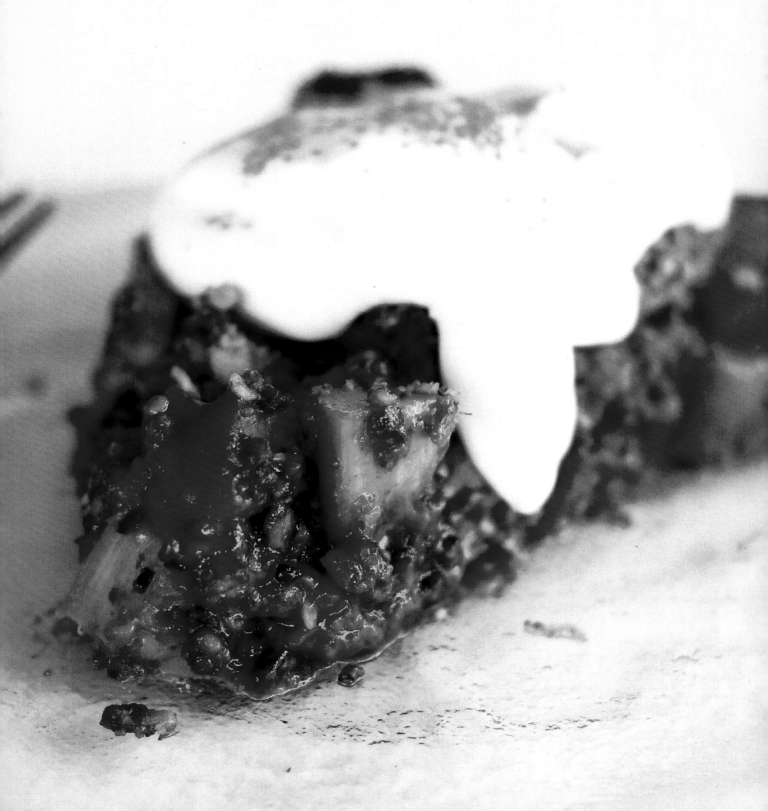

Desserts and Snacks

May have on occasion

Pear Apple Crisp
(Calories: 200, 4 g protein, 4 g fat, 38 g carbohydrates)

Serves 8-10

1	Preheat oven to 400° F	
2	To make filling combine in a 2-quart baking dish all ingredients and set aside.	1 lb. organic apples. thinly sliced 1 lb. organic pears, thinly sliced ½ T. stevia (may use 2 T. maple syrup) 1 t. vanilla extract 1 T. arrowroot powder 1 t. cinnamon ½ C. organic unsweetened apple juice
3	To make the topping mix ingredients well and pour over filling.	½ C. rolled oats ½ C. almond meal ¼ C. coconut oil (liquefied) ¼ t. stevia or 1 T. maple syrup 1 C. toasted walnuts, chopped
4	Cover dish with foil and bake for 45 minutes. Uncover and continue baking until golden brown about 20 minutes.	
5	May be eaten warm or at room temperature.	

Tip: Add topping of yogurt made from the Yogurt Desert recipe.

Energy Cookies
(Calories: 250, 4 g protein, 15 g fat, 24 g carbohydrates)

Makes 18-24 large cookies

1	Preheat oven to 350° F	
2	Mix dry ingredients. Set aside.	2 C. coconut flour (may use spelt four) 2 C. almond meal 1 C. pumpkin seeds 1 C. sesame seeds 1 C. sunflower seeds 2 C. semi-sweet chocolate chips 1 t. salt 4 t. baking powder
3	Mix wet ingredients.	1 C. currants soaked in ½ C. hot water 1 C. coconut oil, heated to liquid 1 C. maple syrup 2 T. vanilla extract
4	Mix wet into dry ingredients. Batter should be stiff yet moist. Use on egg slightly beaten if too dry or crumbly.	1 organic egg, slightly beaten
5	Using a spoon form cookies and place on a cookie sheet. Flatten cookies slightly.	
6	Bake 15 minutes or until golden around the edges.	

Raspberry-Rhubarb Pie
(Calories: 250, 7 g protein, 8 g fat, 40 g carbohydrates)

Serves 6-8

#	Instructions	Ingredients
1	Preheat oven to 350° F	
2	Place tapioca in a coffee grinder or spice grinder; process until finely ground.	2 t. uncooked tapioca
3	Combine tapioca with ingredients in a bowl and let stand 10 minutes.	4½ C. fresh raspberries (about 24 oz.) 3½ C. chopped fresh rhubarb (about 6 stalks) ¼ C. maple syrup (or use 1 T. stevia) ¼ C. cornstarch ¼ C. apple juice 1/8 t. salt
4	To make the crust combine *Berry good cereal, nuts and coconut oil in a food processor and process until paste is formed. Place in the bottom of a lightly oiled pie pan and gently press the dough into the pie dish. Bake 10 minutes.	2 C. *Berry Good Cereal (may use ½ C. sunflower seeds, ½ C. walnuts, ½ C. oats, 1 t. stevia) ½ C. almonds ¼ C. coconut oil liquefied
5	Spoon raspberry mixture into crust and bake 40 minutes.	
6	While pie bakes, combine cereal or nuts, flour and sweetener in a food processor; pulse 10 times until mixture resembles coarse crumbs.	¼ C. Berry Good Cereal or almonds 1 t. stevia or **maple sprinkles 5 T. coconut flour (may use wheat)
7	Increase oven temperature to 375° and sprinkle topping over pie. Bake 15 minutes more. Cool before serving.	

*See resources for Lydia Organic
**Shady Maple Farms from www.citadelle-camp.coop.com

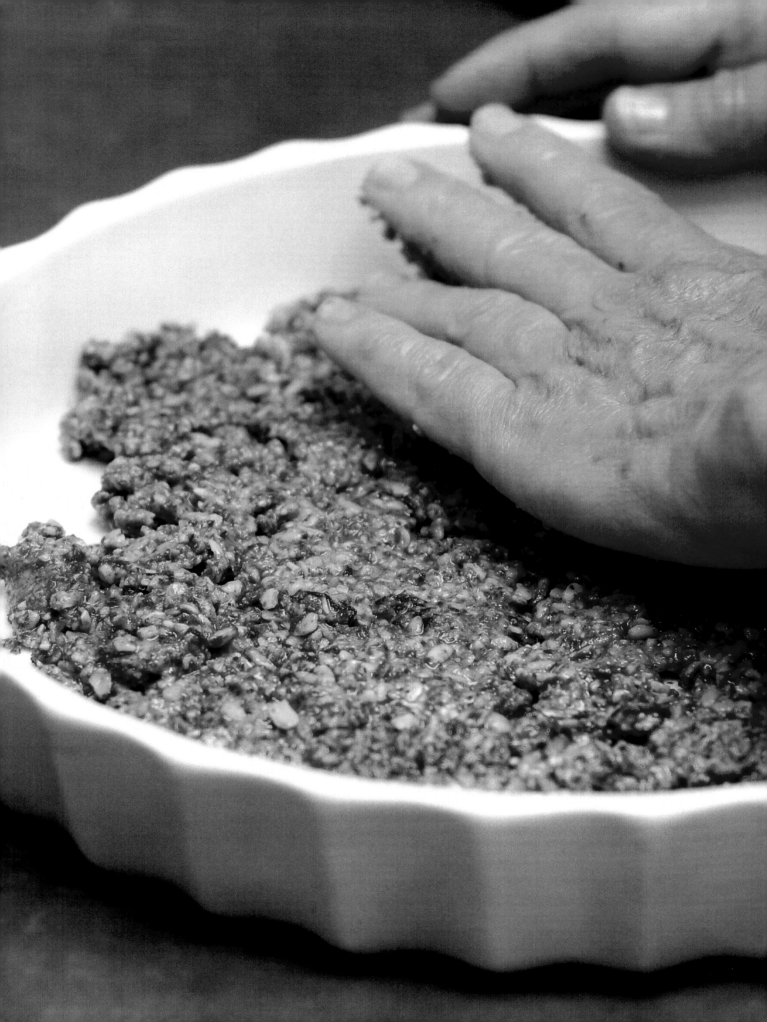

Banana Cashew Slice

(Calories: 120, 2 g protein, 5 g fat, 17 g carbohydrates)

Serves 6-8

1	Preheat oven to 375° F	
2	Blend in food processor or blender.	¼ C. coconut oil, warmed to liquid 2 medium bananas ½ t. vanilla extract 1 t. cinnamon ¼ t. cardamom
3	Add to mixture and blend.	½ C. cashews
4	Add to mixture and blend.	1 C. dry unsweetened coconut flakes ½ C. rolled oats 1 apple, grated
5	Pour into a greased 9 inch baking pan. Bake for 25-30 minutes.	
6	Cool; cut into wedges.	

Tip: Top with yogurt topping and toasted unsweetened coconut flakes.

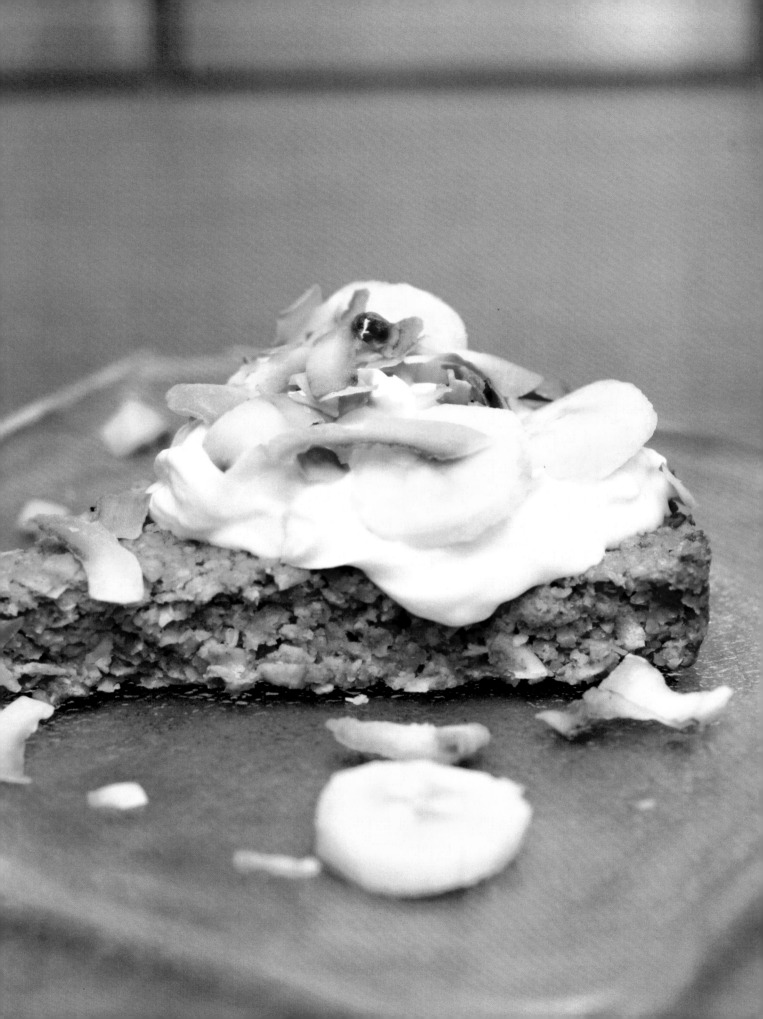

Energy Trail Mix for #2-O

(1/4 cup serving: Calories 200, 9 g protein, 18 g fat, 18 g carbohydrates)

Serves 26

1	In a medium size bowl mix all the ingredients.	½C. dried wild blueberries ½C. coconut flakes, unsweetened 1 C. *coca nibs 1 C. pecans, whole, raw 1 C. peanuts, unsalted 1 C. walnuts 1 C. pumpkin seeds, unsalted
2		May add: ½ t. stevia or maple sprinkles ¼ t. sea salt *cocoa nibs can be used in recipes or for a snack when chocolate taste buds need satisfying. May be found at your health food store.

1. Yogurt Dessert or
2. Ricotta Cheese Dessert

erves 4-6

1	**Yogurt Dessert**	
	In bowl mix yogurt with stevia and vanilla extract until smooth.	15 oz. *Greek plain yogurt (full fat)
		1 T. stevia powder or 2-3 T honey
	In 4-6 custard cups place ½ cup chopped berries top with ½ cup yogurt mixture and sprinkle with ½ T toasted nuts, serve.	1 t. vanilla extract
		½ lb. fresh berries
		½ C. chopped nuts, toasted
2	**Ricotta Dessert**	
	Mix ricotta in bowl with stevia or honey and vanilla.	1 pt. ricotta cheese, full fat
		1 T. stevia or 2-3 T. honey
	Grate the chocolate and gentle fold into cheese mixture.	1 t. vanilla extract
		1 squares 72% dark chocolate
	Place ½ cup in small cup or glass and top with a macaroon cookie.	4-6 macaroon cookies

ip: * Greek style yogurt is strained and thicker similar to sour cream in consistency. Fage brand is widely available or go to www.fageusa.com

Glossary

Arrowroot: A white powder used for thickening sauces. It becomes clear when cooked.

Arugula (Rocket Rugula): An elongated green leaf with a peppery sharp almost mustardy flavor. It can be used in place of spinach in soups and vegetables stews.

Barley: An ancient grain that is very digestible. Hulled barley is superior over pearl barley but it requires longer cooking time and is chewier.

Bragg Liquid Aminos: This is a very tasty soy sauce-like condiment made by extracting amino acids from organic soybeans. It is not fermented, making it an ideal seasoning for those who suffer from yeast sensitivities. You can find it in most health food stores.

Capers: Pickled flower buds. Adds a salty taste; always rinse before using.

Coconut oil: It is a saturated fat that cooks at high temperatures without smoking.

Couscous: A staple of North Africa is made of durum wheat stripped of the bran and germ. Try and get whole wheat couscous which has the bran. It is very quick to cook in less than five minutes.

Curry Paste: A concentrated seasoned mixture of red chilies and spices found in oriental and eastern foods. It can be very hot.

Curry Powder: A blend of spices with degrees of "heat" from maker to maker. Most curry powders have the following: cumin, coriander, mustard seeds, fenugreek, red chilies, black pepper, and turmeric.

Cardamom: A spice found in curry powders. It adds a sweet-spiciness to baked goods and cuts through the flavor and texture of oil.

Fennel: Has a sweet licorice taste. The plant looks like celery. Sliced in salads or soups it adds a delicate taste. I prefer the fennel raw or I like to add at the end of the dish to retain the flavor.

Fish Sauce: Made from salted anchovies. May use in place of salt or soy sauce. It has a very pungent aroma, but the aroma will mellow with cooking.

Flax Seeds: Have a high omega-3 fatty acid ratio and make for a good binder in baked goods. They have a sweet nutty flavor. Because of their high oil content, the seeds tend to go rancid. Store them whole in the freezer for up to three months and grind as needed. They have a laxative effect so eat flax in moderation.

Garam Masala: A blend of dry roasted spices used in Indian cooking. Combination of about twelve spices including: black pepper, cinnamon, cloves, coriander, cumin, fennel, mace and nutmeg. Add towards the end of cooking for more flavors.

Ghee: Clarified butter used in Indian and Middle Eastern cooking. It can be made by melting unsalted butter and removing the scum and foam from the top as it melts.

Ginger, fresh: Buy ginger fresh with smooth skin and store in your refrigerator in a brown bag sealed tightly. To use the root cut a piece and grate or slice. It is not necessary to peel the root unless it is dark brown and shriveled. It should have plenty of juice which can be added to the dish as well. If the recipe calls for fresh ginger you can not substitute dried as it has an entirely different flavor.

Goatein protein powder: A protein powder made from pre-digested goats milk. Made by Garden of Life.

Gomasio: Ground sesame seeds and sea salt.

Great Northern Beans: These are white beans harvested in the Mid-west.

Hemp protein powder: Contains all essential amino acids along with a balance of omega 6 and omega 3 in a ratio of 3 to 1. It also contains GLA for hormone balancing.

Lentils: A very ancient legume. There are many varieties. Brown have a peppery taste, green have a milder taste and my favorite are the French variety that are smaller, sweeter and hold its shape in soups and salads.

Quinoa: Native grain from the Andes and about the size of a sesame seed. Has higher protein and amino acid profile. Be sure and rinse well to remove the bitter saponin coating (believed to be a natural insect repellant) before cooking and drain it thoroughly.

Rhubarb: Considered a fruit it is really a vegetable with red stalks and poisonous leaves. Select medium–thick stalks to slender so they are less stringy; can be stored in the refrigerator for one week sealed in a plastic bag. For cooking rinse well and cut off the ends and slice as directed.

Sea salt: Evaporated seawater which leaves trace minerals lost in refined salt. Has less sodium. Celtic salt is the best quality and can be purchased at Ultra Life (see under resources).

Soba Noodles: Buckwheat noodles. Generally, have other ingredients. I prefer the Eden Foods' brand. The Japanese technique of adding ½ cup of cold water to the boiling water twice during cooking time allows the middle of the noodle to cook thoroughly before the outside becomes soft and mushy.

Spelt: An ancient grain with a texture very similar to wheat. Some people who have sensitivity to wheat may be able to tolerate spelt.

Stevia: Natural sweetener from a plant grown in South America. It is ten times sweeter than sugar so use less.

Tamari: Type of naturally fermented soy sauce that takes a year to ferment. I prefer the organic wheat free type.

Tahini: Sesame butter; a rich peanut-buttery paste used in Middle Eastern and Asian cooking.

Tobasco Sauce: A well known brand name of a hot sauce used in vegetable or meat dishes.

Whey protein powder: Lactose free protein made from cow dairy. Use only good quality without any other ingredients or additives. Ultra Life Whey Natural is a great powder (see resources).

Legends, Weights and Measures

pinch = less then ¼ teaspoon
t.= teaspoon
T.= Tablespoon
C. = Cup
oz. = ounce
pt. = pint
lb. = pound
qt. = quart

To convert to metric

1 Cup = 250 ml
1 Tablespoon = 15 ml (Australia it would be 20 ml)
1 teaspoon = 5 ml

Oven setting equivalents

	Fahrenheit	Celsius	Gas regulo No
Very cool	225-275°	110-140	¼-1
Cool	300-325°	150-160	2-3
Moderate	350-375°	180-190	4-5
Hot	400-450°	200-260	6-8
Very Hot	475-500°	250-260	9-10

Grams to Ounces: These are converted to the nearest round number.

25=1	50=2	75=3	100=3.5	125=4	150=5
175=6	200=7	225=8	250=9	275=10	300=10.5
325=11	350=12	400=14	425=15	450=16	

1 kilogram= 1000 grams= 2lb. 4 oz.

Index

Green Beans with Mushrooms, 50
Cheese and Spinach Stuffed Portobello's, 55

Nuts and Seeds
Energy Trail Mix, 80

Pancakes
Almond Pancakes, 25

Pears
Pear Apple Crisp, 74

Pork
Mini Mushroom and Sausage Quiches, 23
Prosciutto wrapped Asparagus, 48
Bacon-wrapped Pork Tenderloin Filet, 65

Raspberry
Raspberry-Rhubarb Pie, 76
Protein Smoothie, 20

Salads
Artichoke and Ripe Olive with Tuna Salad , 33
Stuffed Artichoke with Hot Crabmeat Salad, 34
Cold Asparagus with Sesame-ginger Vinaigrette, 32

Salmon
Salmon Omelet, 27
Salmon Cakes, 59

Smoothies
Basic berry, 20
Creamy monkey, 20
Reese's pieces, 20
Tropical delight, 20
Raspberry delight, 20

Sausage
Mini Mushroom and Sausage Quiches, 23
Sausage Mushroom Spinach Frittata, 22

Soups
Chicken Bone Broth, 40
Chicken and Spinach, 42
Cleansing Broth, 38
Mushroom Barley and Beef Soup, 44
Salmon Chowder, 41
Split Pea and Ham, 45
Vegetable Broth #2, 40

Vegetables
Green Beans with Mushrooms, 50
Cheesy Cauliflower Bake, 53
Restaurant Green Beans, 51
Blue Cheese-walnut Green Beans. 51
Cheese and spinach Stuffed Portobello's, 55
Broiled Cauliflower, 52
Mashed Cauliflower "Potatoes", 54
Prosciutto Wrapped Asparagus, 45